Reversing the Side Effects of the COVID-19 Vaccine

How to Heal Yourself from Adverse Reactions to the Trump Vaccine and Protect Yourself from Shedding

Mike Stone

Contents

Buyer's Remorse ... 7

The Cause of All Disease ... 12

Juicing—the First Step in Every Healing Program ... 23

Better Out of Your Body than in Your Body ... 29

Emotions and Your Health ... 41

The Amazing Power of Sunlight ... 52

Sleep Like a King ... 55

Honesty is the Best Policy ... 59

Dealing with Depression ... 65

Dealing with Dopes ... 70

My Personal Protection Plan from Shedding ... 73

The Best Advice I Can Give You ... 76

Author contact: mikestone114@yahoo.com

What a World

We live in turbulent times.

Pro-vaccine extremists openly ridicule the unvaxxed and are hysterically vocal in their desire to see them die. What's more, they are giddy with joy in their anticipation of such a thing happening; of seeing half of humanity perish before their eyes.

On the pro-choice side, a tiny minority are equally vocal in their desire to see the vaccinated suffer and die from side effects of the jab. Many of them are just as giddy in their hope to see that happen.

What neither side realizes is that they are both what Vladimir Lenin called "useful idiots," expendable pawns being played on the chess board of life.

This book is intended for reasonable people on both sides; for those who took the jab in good faith and are now experiencing debilitating side effects, and for those who have not taken the jab, but are concerned with the harmful effects of shedding from those who have.

This is a short, easy-to-read book. It's designed that way purposely. I know the desperation one experiences when searching for a cure to an illness that others call incurable and the frustration of spending hours and hours slogging through hundreds of filler pages in poorly-written books looking for that cure. Here, in less than an hour of reading, you'll find all of your answers.

This book is different from any other book you have ever read. I have no product to sell you, no axe to grind, no agenda to get across. My only concern is the truth.

A Quick Word about Shedding

You may have heard stories about how those who have received the COVID-19 vaccine are "shedding" and causing others around them to get sick.

Chief among those shedding stories are numerous reports of unvaccinated pregnant women experiencing miscarriages after spending time around vaccinated people. Indeed, a private school in Florida recently made headlines when, in order to protect the health of their pregnant staff members, they announced that vaccinated teachers were not welcome at their school.

Is it really dangerous for the non-vaccinated to be in close proximity to the vaccinated? At this point, nobody knows for sure, but my experience tells me there is something to it.

Several weeks ago, I made the mistake of ordering food from a restaurant where the entire staff was vaccinated. Within hours I felt ill and dehydrated, and a bump appeared on my head that is still there today.

Coincidence?

More recently, I sat next to a girl on a bus for five minutes. I don't know for certain that she was vaccinated; however, she was wearing two face masks, one on top of the other. What are the odds of someone with that mentality not being vaccinated?

Anyway, I immediately developed a massive headache that lasted over five hours. I also developed an unquenchable need for liquids. In a two hour period, I drank over a gallon of lemon water, organic celery juice and raw milk without urinating once. Like a sponge submerged in a pail of water, my body absorbed every drop.

I didn't feel excessive thirst, but I knew my body needed liquid nourishment, *craved* liquid nourishment. There was something about sitting next to that girl on the bus for five minutes that caused me to experience severe dehydration.

Coincidence?

So, yeah, I do believe there is something to the shedding we've been hearing about. This book provides a wealth of information for those who wish to protect themselves from shedding's harmful effects, including my own personal protocol.

Disclaimer

This work is for informational purposes only, and is not intended to diagnose or treat any disease. The author and publisher present the information, and the reader accepts it, with the understanding that everything done or tried as a result from reading this work is at the reader's own risk. The author and publisher have no liability or responsibility to any person or entity with respect to any loss, damage or injury caused, or alleged to be caused, directly or indirectly by the information contained in this book.

Chapter One

Buyer's Remorse

So you took the jab and now you're feeling remorse. Are you worried about the vaccine's side effects? Are you among the unvaccinated and concerned about shedding from people who have taken the COVID-19 vaccine? You're not alone. There are millions of more people just like you. Unlike the many doom-and-gloomers out there, I do not subscribe to the theory that all is lost, that the ill effects of the Trump vaccine are irreversible; a burden one must carry for the rest of their life.

The reason I don't believe this is because everyone who has studied health and the human body on any level knows that there are natural ways to heal every disease under the sun: cancer of every kind, arthritis, diabetes, degenerative nerve disease, heart disease, gall stones and kidney stones, Alzheimer's, poor vision, and on and on. You name it; there are ways to heal it. Why should the jab be any different? Why should this be the only incurable condition known to man? It's simply not logical.

At this point, nobody knows what is in the Trump vaccine that is making people sick and killing them or what is involved with the shedding that's causing non-vaccinated people to become ill and suffer miscarriages. However, whatever it is can be summed up in one word: toxicity. And the way to remove toxicity from the body is the same no matter what the source.

The body doesn't care where toxicity comes from; it only wants to remove it.

To remove toxicity caused by air pollution requires the same protocol as removing toxicity caused by processed food, or caused by drugs and alcohol, or caused by anything else, including the Trump vaccine and whatever compounds are in the shedding.

With that thought in mind, this book was written.

Inside these pages you will find proven protocols for reversing the damage done by drugs and debilitating disease. You will learn how to cleanse, strengthen and heal your body, how to rebuild your immune system from the ground up and how to return your body to a paradise of vibrant health.

The journey from ill health to good health is simple, but not easy. There are sacrifices you must make and if you aren't willing to make those sacrifices, then there is little chance you will succeed in your quest for wellness.

What kind of sacrifices am I talking about? You can't become healthy on a diet of sugar and junk food. You can't cleanse your body if you continue to pollute it with drugs and alcohol. You can't succeed with a healing protocol while being undermined by toxic friends and family members. All of those things will have to go.

Too much, you say?

Then perhaps this isn't the right book for you.

For every desire, there is a price. The price of good health is the elimination of everything that contributes to poor health. Simple, as I said, but not easy.

In order to truly heal yourself, you're going to have to do the most frightening thing on earth for most people to do: change. And by change I don't mean a little change; I mean huge, cataclysmic changes in every area of your life. Does that worry you?

The fear of change is rampant among humans. It's the reason why so many ninnies and naysayers say natural healing won't work, and why they claim diseases that can be easily healed like cancer and arthritis are "incurable."

They react that way because they are deathly afraid of change. Ask them to change any aspect of their life and they shriek like frightened little girls. "I want my mommy! Wah-wah-wah!"

People like that are happy to swallow a pill or let a complete stranger stick a needle in their arm, but give up their pastries, pies and morning coffee? No way!

Their aversion to change makes healing impossible for them, but that doesn't mean it has to be impossible for *you*. Rather than fear change, embrace it. Look upon change as something fun, something exciting, and then watch the miracle of healing take place in your body.

I know from where I speak, because I was told at a young age that I would be crippled for life, yet I healed myself of "incurable" arthritis. As a child, I was practically blind with astigmatism and vision of 20/800, yet I healed my astigmatism and improved my "incurable" vision to 20/60, and it's still improving.

I've watched and assisted others heal themselves of "incurable" illnesses. I've studied the work of natural healers who have helped hundreds of thousands of people heal their "incurable" diseases. What the world is facing now with the Trump vaccine is no different.

There's a spiritual component to good health also and it might be the most important component of all. We'll cover that near the end of the book, along with the healing power of love and the need to live an honest life. If you've never considered the power of prayer, the power of love, and the power of honesty when it comes to healing the body, you're in for a treat.

This book is not for the weak, the effeminate, or the timid. It's certainly not for the stupid. It's for brave men and women who are on a mission to reclaim their health. It's for courageous individuals who want to reverse the side effects of the COVID-19 vaccine, and for those who are determined to protect themselves and their families from the shedding of others who have taken the jab. It's for anyone who wishes to embark on a journey of health and happiness.

Are you ready to take that journey? Are you ready to distance yourself from the fools and cowards who say it can't be done? Are you ready to reclaim your health and protect your family from sickness and disease? Then gird thy loins and soldier on.

Chapter Two

The Cause of All Disease

There are men and women, many of them gone and forgotten, who discovered long ago how to heal the body of every disease you can name. Though most of them are no longer with us, their work remains.

The good news here is twofold. First, we know that the body can be healed of virtually every disease. It's been proven over and over so many times that the subject is no longer open for debate.

Second, there's no need to reinvent the wheel. These great healers of the past, and a few of the present, have already shown us how to do it. All we need do is study their information and apply it to ourselves.

We can pick out a singular approach that one of them has already pioneered, or we can pick and choose parts from each as we see fit. Best of all, we can apply the common denominators that all of them hold.

Toxicity–Your #1 Enemy

Among those forgotten healers of the past is Doctor J.R. Tilden. Close to a hundred years ago, Dr. Tilden outlined the cause and cure of all disease in his book entitled *Toxemia Explained*.

Toxemia Explained can be summed up in a single sentence: all disease–not some, not a little, but all–is caused by toxicity in the body. Remove the toxicity and the body heals itself.

That's it. That's the whole ballgame. The body is self-healing, self-regulating and self-repairing. Therefore, all that's required in order to achieve vibrant health is to remove the toxicity that's causing the body to be sick and the body will heal itself.

That's wonderful news for those who took the jab and are experiencing harmful side effects. If I were in such a state, I would begin immediately to remove the toxic residue of the vaccine from my body.

It's also good news for those who haven't been vaccinated, but are concerned about shedding from those who are. If I was exposed to a vaccinated person, and I have been, I would begin immediately to remove from my body the toxic residue of that encounter. And just how would I rid my body of that toxic residue, you ask?

The first thing I would do is study the work of Doctor Max Gerson, another forgotten name from the past.

Nourish First, Then Detoxify

Dr. Max Gerson was a Jewish physician who left Germany for New York in the 1930s. He was also a medical genius who discovered a way to reverse cancer through a two-pronged approach of juicing and coffee enemas. His motto was "nourish first, then detoxify."

Dr. Gerson's patients first nourished their bodies via fresh, organic fruit, vegetable and liver juices, and then detoxified with coffee enemas.

To the betterment of mankind, Dr. Gerson's program was a tremendous success. Thousands of terminal cancer patients, on their death beds and given up to die, healed themselves by following the Gerson Therapy.

Dr. Gerson's use of coffee enemas to cleanse the liver is dismissed by the ignorant, but it has a long and successful track record of medical application dating back to World War I, when it was used in place of morphine.

Indeed, coffee enemas are universally acknowledged as the greatest pain relief medication in the world and they are an effective treatment for depression. They stimulate the liver to release toxins in the most efficient way known to man.

Dr. Gerson discovered on his own the same thing that Dr. Tilden did: toxicity is the cause of all disease. Said the good doctor, "A patient is unlikely to die from cancer, but from the toxins accumulated in the body."

This is more good news for vaccine sufferers and for anyone worried about shedding. If cancer patients, sick, emaciated and given up for dead, can heal their bodies, then anyone can.

After all, if the adverse side effects of the jab and the resultant shedding are caused by toxic residue, then by removing that toxicity the body will heal.

The Eternal Search for Man's Perfect Diet

Is there an ideal diet for mankind? Specific foods or a method of eating that provides the optimum in health and vitality? Yes, there is, and it was discovered in the 1930s by another forgotten name from the past: Doctor Weston Price.

Dr. Price was a dentist who traveled around the world in the 1930s, studying the teeth and general health of indigenous people. What he found was startling: indigenous people, eating a natural diet with no processed food at all, along with generous portions of raw meat, raw seafood, or raw milk and dairy products, had excellent teeth and dental health, along with strong, physically fit bodies. Dr. Price classified them as almost perfect human specimens.

They had no cancer, no heart disease, no arthritis, none of the diseases that plague modern society. Many of their communities had no police department or jail. There was no need for them; crime did not exist. However, when these same people began eating processed food, brought in by explorers and settlers, everything changed.

Their health deteriorated rapidly. Cancer, heart disease, arthritis, and other illnesses that had been non-existent before, instantly appeared, and crime was now a problem. The same food that most Americans consume on a daily basis destroyed these people.

Dr. Price wrote of his findings in a marvelous book called *Nutrition and Physical Degeneration*. If you want a strong, pain-free body, then one of the best pieces of advice I can give you is to read Dr. Price's book and follow his diet recommendations. There's only one problem. The book is extremely long and makes for pretty stiff reading.

A more efficient way to absorb Dr. Price's research is to go online, do a search for his name, and visit the various websites dedicated to him, such as www.price-pottenger.org and www.westonaprice.org.

You can also learn about Dr. Price and his work by reading the book *Cure Tooth Decay* by Ramiel Nagel. It's an excellent summary of Dr. Price's work and it's extremely easy to read. Everything that book says about eating to improve your teeth also applies to the entire body. In fact, it applies to every illness.

This is more fantastic news for vaccine sufferers or those worried about shedding. You now have a proven resource to consult for just about any dietary question you have.

Liver—Nature's Super Food

Doctor Nicholas Gonzalez is another healer from the past who had great success in reversing cancer and other illnesses. Dr. Gonzalez specialized in pancreatic cancer and part of his protocol was to prescribe raw liver to all of his patients.

Beef liver from grass-fed animals is nature's super food, the most nutritious food on the planet. Raw liver from clean sources and frozen for at least two weeks can restore energy and vitality to even the most exhausted organism.

Liver also has an anti-fatigue factor that no other food possesses. It contains more nutrients, gram for gram, than any other food.

You might not like the taste of liver—I didn't, at first—but once you get used to it, it is absolutely delicious. I buy frozen liver from grass-fed animals at Whole Foods. You can probably find a source where you live.

Herbs for You and Me

Doctor Richard Schulze is yet another giant in the field of health who discovered that all illness is caused by toxicity in the body. Unlike the others we've covered so far, Dr. Schulze is alive and kicking. His healing protocol consists of herbs, juicing, a vegetarian diet, and bowel cleansing. Heavy-duty bowel cleansing.

If you would like to use herbs as part of your healing protocol, Dr. Schulze is your go-to guy. I can personally vouch for the strength and effectiveness of his Echinacea and Anti-I formulas. For anyone concerned about shedding from the vaccine, Echinacea could prove very useful. I took a ton of it after my first encounter with shedding.

Echinacea is one of the strongest immune stimulators we have. It can double or even triple the amount of T-cells in the blood, and offers great protection from potential illness.

Don't discount the power of herbs to heal and rejuvenate the body. They can literally save your life. For instance, did you know that cayenne pepper can literally stop a heart attack in its tracks? It can, and with so many vaccinated people falling ill with blood clots and other heart ailments, herbs are an area that anyone suffering from vaccine related side effects should immediately explore.

Dick Quinn wrote an entire book about the power of cayenne pepper entitled *Left For Dead*. Cayenne pepper saved his life. He used it to heal himself after suffering a near-fatal heart attack and then passed his knowledge on to others.

Quinn researched the healing qualities of cayenne pepper by reading the work of Doctor John Christopher, another great healer of the past.

Herbs are powerful healers. If you've tried them before and weren't satisfied with the results, then it's likely because the herbs you used were too weak.

One Size Fits All

We've now covered four doctors (five, if you include Dr. Christopher) who each discovered independently of each other that toxicity in the body is the cause of all disease. We could list dozens more, but for our purposes these four are sufficient.

These four doctors unanimously agree that the way to heal a toxic body is through a dual process of cleansing and nourishing.

What's more, they all insist that healing protocols are not disease specific. In other words, you don't do this one thing for cancer, and this other thing for heart disease, and a third thing for arthritis. You do the same protocol for every disease every time. Cleansing and nourishing the body works on everyone for everything.

Everything, you say? Yes, everything. Every single disease ever recorded has been healed through cleansing and nourishment, not just once but many times.

19

Your mission, should you decide to accept it, is to create a lifestyle so filled with health and vitality that your body has no choice but to heal itself. A lifestyle filled with nourishment; a lifestyle filled with cleansing and detoxification, a lifestyle filled with positive emotions and life-affirming choices.

If every day of your life is filled with life-affirming choices then your body must heal. In fact, healing is the only option. It's inconceivable for a body continuously nourished and cleansed to remain sick or even to become sick in the first place. Anyone who tells you otherwise is a fool, a liar, or both.

Break down the word "incurable" and what do you get? You get *in*-curable. That means one must go with-*in* to find the cure.

There is no faster way to go with-*in* the body than a program of cleansing and nourishing. It's worked without fail in the past, and it continues to work without fail today.

You can pick a specific protocol from any of the above four doctors, or you can pick and choose parts from each.

Some protocols are harder than others. The Gerson Therapy is probably the hardest, but then it's also one of the most effective with a long history of success. Through trial and error you can discover the one that's right for you.

Your personal healing can proceed as fast or as slow as you desire. You can begin with baby steps if you want. That's perfectly fine.

Just be aware that your progress will be slower and less dramatic. With the four doctors profiled above, most of the people that came to them for healing were knocking on death's door. They couldn't afford to proceed slowly. Their bodies demanded fast and radical change.

When I was crippled from arthritis and unable to move my arm, the pain was so unbearable I couldn't tolerate a slow start. I was forced by necessity to plunge right in and heal myself as quickly as possible.

In the case of improving my vision, there was no pain involved and it wasn't a life or death situation. Therefore, my healing has been more gradual. Although in the last two weeks it has accelerated immensely. I'll talk about why that has occurred that in a future chapter.

Through the remainder of this book, we'll cover some very important steps that are common to just about every healing protocol, including a few new steps that I guarantee you have never heard anywhere else. Consider them my personal gift to you.

Now that you're acquainted with the cause and healing of all disease, ask yourself if there is any reason, any reason at all, why you can't heal your own body from the side effects of the Trump vaccine, or protect your body from the shedding that's coming from those who have taken the jab?

The answer is obvious.

Cleansing your body of toxicity and nourishing it with vitamins, minerals, phytonutrients, sunlight, rest, positive emotions and other essential protocols will heal your body of any illness.

If you're feeling excited right now then you are a prime candidate for success. You should not have any problems in healing your body. Turn the page and get started on the path to wellness.

Chapter Three

Juicing–the First Step in Every Healing Program

Juicing is the first step in any healing program. Why? Because it works.

A sick body needs nutrients in order to get well. It needs those nutrients in large quantities and in a form that's easily assimilated. Juicing covers both bases.

When I talk about juicing, I'm referring to juice you make at home with your own juicer, not any kind of bottled juice available in a store. I'm also talking about organic juice. Pesticide-laden produce is not allowed.

When you juice in this manner you absorb immense quantities of vitamins and minerals in their most easily assimilated form. As a way to nourish a sick body—or as a means of prevention to keep a body from getting sick—juicing has no equal.

Juicing will cleanse toxicity from your body, while simultaneously providing it with a massive influx of easily digestible vitamins, minerals and live enzymes. It's the quickest way possible to super-charge your body with massive nourishment.

Juicing will give you healthier, more vibrant-looking hair, radiant skin, and stronger nails. Who wouldn't want any of those things?

When you juice, you flood your body with first-class, easily-absorbable, nutrient-dense nourishment.

Consuming large quantities of fresh, organic vegetable juice is the fastest, easiest, and most effective way to transform both your health and your appearance.

I've seen men and women of all ages with haggard-looking skin, weary from life and all of its challenges, begin a serious juicing routine and become so beautiful they were almost unrecognizable.

I've seen dull eyes regain their sparkle, gray hair restored to its original color, and pasty skin rebound with a healthy glow. I've seen people who juice, and others of the same age who opt for plastic surgery, and the juicers look ten to twenty years younger than the face-lifters at a fraction of the cost.

Have you ever noticed the beauty and vibrancy of fruits and vegetables; their bright colors, intoxicating scents, and pulsing life? When you juice, you partake of all the healing qualities and all the phytonutrients that God bestowed upon nature.

How can that not reflect itself back in the health and beauty of your own skin?

Fresh juice is a natural blood-builder. There is nothing, absolutely nothing, you can do to improve your health faster and more efficiently than juicing.

When that first sip of mineral-rich juice touches your lips, you'll feel a jolt in every cell of your body. The nutrient-dense, life-creating enzymes will saturate your body and light up your cells with vitality and life.

When you juice, you're building health and beauty from the inside out. When you juice, you separate the mineral elements from the fiber, leaving only liquid nourishment that your body digests almost instantly.

If I was ill from any disease, the first thing I would do is begin drinking large quantities of raw, organic vegetable juice. Indeed, when exposed to vaccinated individuals, the first thing I do is start drinking large quantities of fresh, organic juice in order to flush out the toxins of shedding.

How important is juicing? Doctor Norman Walker says, "Vegetable juices are the builders and regenerators of the body. They contain all the amino acids, minerals, salts, enzymes, and vitamins needed by the human body, provided they are used fresh, raw, and without preservatives."

How important is juicing? Dr. Richard Schulze says, "Sell your television. Sell your furniture and sit on the floor. Sell your car and walk. Sell your clothes. But don't live another day without a juicer."

Feeling depressed? Juicing will snap you right out of it. It is impossible to feel any kind of negative emotion when you flood your body with oxygen-rich nutrients from delicious vegetable juice.

Want more energy? Juicing will give it to you. Once you start, you'll wonder how you ever got along without it. In his book *There Are No Incurable Diseases*, Dr. Richard Schulze writes about being on the 28th day of a 30-day juice fast and kick-boxing for 17 three-minute rounds, a personal best for him. Afterwards, one of the gym's top instructors told Dr. Schulze he was moving so fast he was like a blur.

(Note: Don't attempt a 30-day juice fast unless and until you are very experienced with juicing!)

Juice carrots, celery, cucumbers, lettuce and bell peppers of all colors. Juice cruciferous vegetables like broccoli and cauliflower. Juice carrots and dandelion together. Juice some apples with a slice of lemon and a pinch of ginger. One of the joys of juicing is discovering different combinations to drink. My favorites are celery and cucumber, each juiced separately.

In his book *Life-Changing Foods*, Anthony William calls cucumber juice the best rejuvenation tonic in the world. He says juicing cucumbers unleashes a magical anti-fever element that helps calm a fever like water on a fire, and that drinking 16 ounces of pure cucumber juice on a regular basis, can have a life-changing effect.

If that doesn't make you want to drink a tall, cold glass of cucumber juice, nothing will.

I spoke earlier of the dehydration I experienced from vaccinated people who were shedding. Well, consuming massive amounts of cucumber juice is an easy and effective way to combat that.

No matter what your ailment, if you want a secret weapon to help heal your body, start juicing today.

Juicing doesn't have to be expensive. It can be, but it doesn't have to be. I use a Hamilton Beach juicer, model number 67608Z, that I bought for less than fifty bucks. Other companies have their own inexpensive models.

Of course, if price is no object, the Rolls Royce of juicers is the Norwalk Juice and Press Machine, named after Norman Walker, whom we quoted earlier. It's costly, well over a thousand dollars, but it is the best.

As the world's biggest tightwad, I would never spend that kind of money. But then I'm not rich and I'm not suffering from serious illness. If I were, I wouldn't hesitate to get the best juicer I could find.

The Champion Juicer with a separate press machine is also very good. It's not as costly as the Norwalk Juicer, but it's not cheap either. It will set you back $800.

Are there any drawbacks to juicing, any at all?

Only one I can think of: juicing will increase your need to urinate. For that reason, I wouldn't advise doing it before any type of social event.

However, there's no reason why you can't do it when you are home.

A pleasant side effect of juicing is the way it will beautify your appearance. I guarantee you people will begin to notice and compliment you on your new, healthy-looking skin. If you're single, you may not be single for long. If you're married, your spouse will fall in love with you all over again. I don't care how sick you are or how unattractive you think you might be, juicing will heal and beautify you simultaneously.

For anyone suffering adverse side effects from the Trump vaccine, or from the shedding of vaccinated individuals, juicing is an absolute must.

Have I convinced you of the importance of juicing? It's helped me tremendously. It's helped everyone who has ever tried it. Chances are it will help you too.

Chapter Four

Better Out of Your Body than in Your Body

Now that you've begun to nourish your body with large quantities of fresh, organic juice, the next step is to cleanse it of toxicity. Removal of toxicity is a vital component in restoring health to the body.

If you're intrigued by the Gerson Therapy and its use of coffee enemas for stimulating the liver to release toxins, you can read about the correct procedure for doing them in the books *Healing the Gerson Way* and *The Gerson Therapy*.

As previously noted, coffee enemas, done in the manner that Dr. Gerson prescribed them, are universally acknowledged as the best pain relief medication in the world, and an effective treatment for depression.

Another vital component to cleansing the body is the elimination of all processed food.

Processed food and beverages contain chemicals, pesticides, and preservatives. These are all foreign and toxic to your body. The moment you ingest a foreign substance, your body begins to immediately expel it in whatever way it can. To the uniformed, that elimination process appears as a symptom of sickness.

Think about it. When the body is overloaded with toxicity, it reacts by forcing the toxicity out. If that cannot be accomplished in the usual way—by sweating or going to the bathroom—then the body is forced to do it through other means. The result is a headache, a skin rash, a fever, a tumor, heart palpitations, and on and on.

Those are all symptoms of a toxic body that is straining to heal itself. With this knowledge, you can now see that the common cold is nothing more than your body expelling toxicity. That's why no one has ever discovered a "cure" for the common cold. The cold itself is the cure. It's your body's way of releasing toxins.

Ignorance on this issue is what sends millions of Americans running to their "doctor" for a pill or a shot. However, the pill or the shot only add to the problem by filling the body with more toxicity.

This is eye-opening information for most people and you can judge their knowledge of science, medicine and the body, as well as their ability to heal themselves by their reaction to it. The pencil-necked ninnies we spoke of earlier, the ones that cry for their mommy when confronted with change react the same way with this issue, because it challenges them to change their thinking. And they are frightened to death of change.

Rather than face reality, they shriek and howl and bring up the long-debunked germ theory. Such people will never evolve. Nor will they ever heal themselves of sickness.

On the other hand, those that do see the light, heal themselves very rapidly.

If I were experiencing adverse side effects from the Trump vaccine or from exposure to shedding, I would immediately remove all processed food from my diet. That means anything that comes in a bag, box, can, jar, bottle, or wrapper.

I would also adhere to the following:

No fast food, junk food, or restaurant food.

No non-organic fruits or vegetables; nothing that has been sprayed with pesticides.

No pasteurized dairy products.

No bread, sandwiches or sandwich meat.

No hamburgers. No French fries. No hot dogs.

No pizza. No cereal. No white flour of any sort.

No coffee. No tea. No soda or soft drinks.

No cookies. No cake. No ice cream.

No snack foods. No gum. No candy.

No seedless fruit except bananas.

No jelly. No mustard or ketchup.

No microwaved food.

No tap water—not for drinking, not for cooking, not for brushing my teeth. I would use distilled water only.

No aluminum cookware, only stainless steel.

No drugs, lotions or creams.

No sunscreen. No sunglasses.

No toothpaste that contains fluoride. (Fluoride is an extremely harmful substance.)

No sugar.

No ketchup. No mustard. No condiments of any kind.

No energy bars. No protein bars or protein powders.

That's a pretty extensive list and you might be thinking there's no way that you could follow it.

I'm here to tell you that you can follow it and there's no harm in at least trying it. If you give up now, you are a quitter. Quitters never win, and winners never quit.

What's more, I believe you can do it. I have faith in you, and I'm here to walk with you every step of the way. You can email me for support at any time. You can ask me any question you have. I'm here to help you.

The human body was not designed to consume any of the items listed above. Remember what we said earlier about your body needing to eliminate toxic substances? When you consume the items listed above you force your body to expel the chemicals, pesticides, and preservatives they contain. Now add to that the additional toxicity in your body from the jab or from exposure to shedding. That's a tremendous burden for your body to carry.

Here's an analogy for you. Suppose you were standing in the center of a hole that you were digging and wondering how you will ever get out. Well, the first step in getting out of that hole is to put the shovel down and stop digging.

Similarly, the first step in eliminating toxicity and allowing yourself to heal is to stop putting toxic chemicals, pesticides, and preservatives into your body. Makes sense, doesn't it?

Eliminating the products listed above is a big first step in healing your body. A *huge* first step. What's more, it's not hard or unpleasant. The truth is once you begin eliminating unhealthy food from your life and replace it with healthy food you will love the taste. You will love it so much you will never go back to processed food again. I guarantee it.

You haven't lived until you've eaten a slice of cold watermelon with seeds, or taken a bite from a perfectly ripe banana with little brown spots on the peel, or eaten an ice-cold chilled cherimoya, otherwise known as the ice cream fruit. (Yes, it is a fruit and, yes, it does taste like ice cream.)

Wild salmon eaten raw or grilled and served with vegetables and/or a salad is absolutely delicious. Beef from grass-fed animals tastes amazing. Raw milk with some raw cream mixed in tastes so good it's almost impossible to stop drinking. (Unfortunately, it's also hard to find unless you live in California.)

Here's what you can eat and drink: wild, ocean-caught salmon and tuna (not canned), meat from grass-fed animals, organically grown fruits and vegetables (make sure your fruit contains seeds), raw milk and dairy products (available in only a handful of states, so you're probably out of luck), distilled water with organic lemon juice squeezed in, homemade vegetable and fruit juices made with organic produce. And don't forget all that delicious juice you're going to consume.

The list of allowable foods is small compared to the not-allowable list, but within it is infinite variety. And within that list are nutritionally rich foods that will heal, strengthen, and beautify your body. Instead of overloading it with toxicity, you will be flooding your body with rich, blood-building nutrition.

If you're wondering where to get wild, ocean-caught fish, grass-fed meat, organic produce, and the rest, try your local grocery store. They might surprise you. Farmer's markets are another choice; most communities have them. Health food stores are also an option.

When buying produce, look at the numbered sticker. If it's a five-digit number, beginning with the number 9, then that produce is organic. That's what you want.

If you see a four-digit number, beginning with the number 4, then that produce is conventional, which means it was grown with pesticides. That's what you don't want.

If you see a five-digit number, beginning with the number 8, then that produce is Genetically Modified. That's what you absolutely do not want, under any circumstances.

Almost all potatoes today are GMO. So never eat restaurant potatoes, and never buy or eat potatoes unless you know for a fact that they are organic.

Now if you're really strapped, if you live out in the boondocks and literally have no sources for organic produce, then—and only then—you will have to make do with what you have. In other words, you will have to settle for produce that is not organic. But make sure you soak and wash it to remove as much pesticide as possible. One way to do that is to add a quarter cup of 3% food-grade hydrogen peroxide to a gallon of cold water and soak your produce in it. For leafy vegetables, 15-20 minutes should be enough. For thick-skinned fruits and vegetables, soak them for 30-35 minutes.

Soaking non-organic produce is not the preferable approach, but if that's your only option, go ahead and do it.

Conventional produce with peels, like bananas and oranges, are not as bad as conventional produce without peels, like apples and grapes. I eat conventional Dole bananas on occasion, as well as conventional avocadoes and conventional broccoli that has been well rinsed or soaked. But they're never my first choice. If you're on a quest to heal your body, you may want to avoid them.

All of this is going to take a little effort on your part. It's not always easy to find healthy sources of food, but it can be done. If you live with others and they aren't willing to help, you'll simply have to do it on your own. After all, it's your health, not theirs.

You can try explaining to them how the body is self-healing and why you need to avoid processed food and only consume organic produce, ocean-caught fish, meat from grass-fed animals, and distilled water in order to heal yourself. But don't be surprised if it falls on deaf ears. Most people are unwilling to listen to logic.

The bottom line regarding other people is if they are willing to help you, fantastic. If not, that's fantastic too. You can look on the situation as a marvelous opportunity to become self-sufficient. That alone will put you ahead of the majority of people in the world.

If you're feeling discouraged because you don't think you will be able to eliminate processed food from your diet, take heart. You can do it. Others, with far less going for themselves than you, have done it. If they can do it, then so can you.

What's important right now is that you take the first step. Clean out your kitchen and stock it up with the delicious healing foods we've discussed. Throw that processed swill into the trash where it belongs. Don't even give it away.

Distilled Water

The reason for using distilled water is the same as avoiding processed food. Tap water and most brands of bottled water contain fluoride and other chemicals. You don't want fluoride or other chemicals anywhere in or on your body. So use distilled water only to brush your teeth and wash your face. Put some into a little spray bottle and spray it on your face or on your toothbrush. For guys, use distilled water for shaving, and avoid shaving cream. Use distilled water only or natural soap with no chemicals to shave your face.

You can squeeze some organic lemon juice into distilled water for drinking. And always use distilled water for cooking, never use tap water. Almost every drugstore and grocery store in the country sells distilled water.

Practice Proper Food Combining

Practice proper food combining when eating. Protein, starches, and fruit require different enzymes in order to digest properly. For that reason, consume fruits or fruit juice alone, at least one hour before consuming any other type of food. Two hours before is better.

Consume starches alone, although ideally you should avoid all starches, except organic yams. You can eat protein, such as meat or fish, with vegetables, but not with fruits or starches. The lone exception might be organic potatoes mixed in with beef stew. Consume vegetable juice alone. Consume dairy products alone.

If you ignore proper food combining, your body will have great difficulty digesting your meals. If that happens, you've just created more toxicity in your body, and you know what the next step is, right? Your body will begin releasing that toxicity in whatever way it can.

Don't drink liquid with meals. Drinking liquid with meals causes bloating and makes it hard for your body to digest your food. Instead, drink between meals. Drink distilled water with organic lemon juice squeezed in at least three hours after a meal, and at least 30 minutes before a meal. And drink a lot of water. It will help your body flush out toxicity.

Eat slowly and sip your liquids. This is important. Slow eating means a lot of chewing, as well as putting your fork down between bites. This will make it a lot easier for your body to digest what you are consuming. If you shovel food into your mouth and swallow it down, your digestion will be severely impaired. Sadly, that's the way most people eat.

Sip your liquids slowly for the same reason, especially when drinking juice.

Whether eating or drinking, relax and think pleasant thoughts. If you're tense or excited, you make it hard for your body to digest food.

What about supplements, you ask? There are only two that I recommend: Vitamin C powder from organic food sources, such as acerola cherry, and fermented cod liver oil with X Factor Gold Concentrated Butter Oil.

If you can't afford those items, don't worry. They're helpful, but not necessary. I didn't have them when I healed myself of "incurable" arthritis, and I don't think I would have healed myself any faster if I did have them.

We're less than halfway through this book, but you already have plenty of information to begin healing yourself from any type of adverse reaction to the Trump vaccine or from the effects of shedding. The bottom line is to eat *real* food in a calm and tranquil setting, and avoid any and all processed food, plus plenty of juicing. With these steps alone, you're well on your way to a healthy body. You *can* do it.

When I healed my arthritis–and my arthritis was *bad,* two doctors told me it was the worst case they had ever seen and that I would be crippled for life–I had less information than you have now. But I healed myself completely by changing what I was eating and drinking. There's no reason why you can't do the same. Remember the basics:

All disease is caused by toxicity in the body.

Your situation is no different.

All reputable doctors and health professionals agree that the way to eliminate illness is to eliminate toxicity from the body.

Your situation is no different.

All reputable doctors and health professionals agree that nourishing the body through proper nutrition is the first step in healing the body of any disease.

Your situation is no different.

All reputable doctors and health professionals agree that detoxifying the body is the second step in healing the body of any disease.

Your situation is no different.

All reputable doctors and health professionals agree that junk food, processed food, cigarettes, drugs and alcohol should be avoided in order to have a healthy, disease-free body. Your situation is no different.

Now let's look at the role that emotions play when it comes to healing.

Chapter Five

Emotions and Your Health

Earlier in this book we talked about hatred; seething, foaming-at-the-mouth hatred that pro-vax extremists have for the unvaxxed.

Where does all that hatred come from? The answer is simple: it comes from self-hatred. It's impossible to hate someone else without hating yourself first.

Some people call self-hatred a form of demon possession and I wouldn't disagree with them. Self-hatred *is* very often a sign of possession.

The Bible tells us to love God with our whole mind, heart, body and soul, and to love our neighbor as ourselves. A person wrapped in self-hatred can do neither of those things.

When a crowd of self-hating individuals get together, the result is what we saw throughout the year 2020 and that we continue to see today in places like Portland: rioting and looting on a mass scale. The people that participate in such activities, as well as those that support them, are combustible caricatures of self-hatred. And many of them do appear to be under a form of possession.

For our purposes it's important to note that self-hating people rarely enjoy good health, and that love, which is the opposite of hate, is a necessary step in the process of self-healing. Without love, your odds of succeeding are slim.

What the Wise Have Always Known

Are you aware of the immense role that emotions play in your health? Every emotion we experience corresponds to a specific organ in the body. It's something the ancients have always known. It's only in the last one hundred years or so that we've forgotten.

Have you ever heard the expression "green with envy"? That expression is hundreds of years old. It comes from the fact that envy corresponds to the gallbladder, which is green in color. When a person experiences envy, they weaken their gallbladder.

Have you ever heard someone say, "I was so angry I couldn't see straight" or "I was so mad I saw red"? That's because anger corresponds to the liver, which is red in color and affects the vision. Almost all vision problems originate in childhood trauma related to anger. The child sees or experiences something that is so disturbing he literally distorts his vision in order to block it from sight.

That doesn't mean the child was abused, necessarily. He may have lost a pet, or watched something violent on television, or had a disturbing experience at school.

If you wear glasses or contact lenses, think back to when you first began wearing them.

Did you experience some sort of emotional upheaval at the time? Was there something going on in your life—arguing or fighting between your parents, perhaps, or something similar—that you didn't want to see?

I would bet money that the answer is yes.

In addition to its effect on vision, anger can cause a person's skin to erupt in rashes or acne (also red in color).

Old time physicians were much more attuned to the relationship between emotions and health than today's drug pushers. In the old days sick and diseased people were often sent to sanitariums out in the country. In those tranquil settings, far from the hustle and bustle of city life and its daily problems, their bodies had a chance to rest and recuperate.

If we still did that today, many people would heal themselves of many different illnesses. Instead, they're drugged up and sent home to die.

Stress can turn hair gray and cause premature aging. If you have ever seen photographs of presidents before and after their time in office, the difference is startling. The enormous pressure and responsibility of holding that office (and consequently lying on a daily basis) takes an enormous toll on their appearance. Throw in the fact that almost all of them were corrupt and evil men to begin with and it's no wonder that so many of them appear to have aged markedly during only four to eight years in office. The lone exceptions appear to be Ronald Reagan and Donald Trump.

Pushed to the extreme, negative emotions can be fatal. Sudden shock or fright can cause a heart attack and actually kill a person.

Just as negative emotions have a debilitating effect on the body and create toxicity, positive emotions have an uplifting effect on the body and contribute to good health.

One famous case involves the writer Norman Cousins. He was diagnosed with cancer and cured himself with laughter. Yes, you read that right. He literally laughed his way to health by using humor to cure his cancer.

Cousins knew that negative emotions were contributing to his cancer, so he began watching old comedy movies. Hours of them. He spent his days laughing, which stimulated his immune system, and very soon his cancer was gone. It was so extraordinary he wrote a book about it called *Anatomy of An Illness*.

Louise Hay is another author who healed her illness with positive emotions. Like Cousins, she was diagnosed with cancer and set out to heal herself. Louise didn't use laughter like Cousins did, but she did use positive emotions, positive affirmations, and positive thinking as the basis for her therapy. Like Cousins, she succeeded in completely healing her cancer. Like Cousins, she also wrote a book called *You Can Heal Your Life.*

(Note: while both of these authors are admirable for the self-healing work they did, I do not recommend reading either of their books. That's because in addition to the healing advice they contain, they also allude to and contain false and detrimental spiritual advice. I mention the titles here for reference only.)

Emotions not only affect our health, they also affect our appearance. Bitter, angry, and resentful people often age more rapidly than others. Their stored up anger and overwhelms the function of their liver and other organs and their skin takes on a sick and sallow complexion.

On the other hand, those who practice forgiveness and cultivate positive emotions often retain a youthful appearance well into middle age and beyond. Amazing isn't it?

It's said that you can predict how a person will look in twenty years' time by seeing their face after they run a marathon. I think a far better method is to view a person when angry; to witness their angry and bitter facial contortions vs. the glowing cheeks and sparkle in the eye of a happy and joyous person. Those are much more accurate ways to predict how a person will look twenty years later.

Laugh and the World Laughs With You

As we saw with Norman Cousins, humor is very healing.

Did you know that it's impossible to feel anger towards a person with whom you've just shared a laugh?

It's true. If there's someone in your life you can't stand, try telling them a joke the next time you see them. That smirk of laughter your words manage to evoke could go a long way towards healing your relationship with that person.

I recommend you get your hands on a good joke book (a *good* joke book, I said, not a stupid one), pick out a dozen or so of the funniest jokes, and memorize them. Then start using them. You can also find jokes for free on the internet and you can make up your own. I make up a lot of my own jokes.

Unfortunately, I can't recommend any funny movies or comedians, because none of them are funny.

Keep your jokes clean. The laughter you bring out in others and experience for yourself will help heal your body.

If there are children in your life, pick up a joke book for kids. Kids *love* jokes. Their laughter and smiles and will bring out the laughter and smiles in you.

In addition to humor, you will find it good for your health to engage in positive thoughts. If someone has wronged you in the past (or in the present), forgive that person. That doesn't mean forgoing justice. If a person has committed a crime against you, it's important that you continue to seek justice and perhaps jail time for that person. Those responsible for orchestrating the virus hoax need to be held accountable. But don't hold a grudge.

Forgive everyone from your past, including and especially the person you find it most difficult to forgive. Your forgiveness of that person is necessary for your own healing.

When you refuse to forgive someone, you're basically allowing that person to continue to harm you. Think about that. Why would you want to continue to experience pain from someone in your past? Forgive and let go. But don't forget, lest you get hurt again.

Forgiveness and focusing on positive thoughts does not mean you will never experience anger. In fact, anger is a necessary emotion. You want to feel anger when you witness injustice and especially when confronted with evil. Psalm 97 says, "Ye that love the LORD hate evil." That's one of the most important sentences in the entire Bible. It describes good righteous anger.

Saint Thomas Aquinas, one of the wisest men in the history of the world, said, "He who is not angry when there is just cause for anger is immoral. Why? Because anger looks to the good of justice. And if you can live amid injustice without anger, you are immoral as well as unjust."

Saint John Chrysostom, another great wise man, said, "He who is not angry, whereas he has cause to be, sins. For

47

unreasonable patience is the hotbed of many vices, it fosters negligence, and incites not only the wicked but even the good to do wrong."

So forgive the person who borrowed your favorite book and never returned it, forgive the person who stole the girl or guy you liked, forgive the person who wronged you and the person in your life that you can't stand being around the most. But continue to hold righteous, indignant anger against the sins of man.

It's okay to feel righteous anger at the murder of babies by abortion.

It's okay to feel righteous anger at the non-stop lies coming from Hollywood and the mainstream media.

It's okay to feel righteous anger at the corruption of so many who hold political office.

It's okay to feel righteous anger at unjust wars, both military and economic.

It's okay to feel righteous anger at the actions of those who seek to destroy the family, those who seek to destroy the country by rioting, looting, and burning down cities, and those who seek to topple Christianity.

You get the idea.

Now what if you're feeling anger right now, not at the injustices I detailed above, but because you support those things? If that's the case, I want you to hold on to your anger for a moment and ask yourself who in your life you are most angry with.

You might get only a vague, general feeling, but keep asking yourself that question and see if you can personalize it. Most likely someone will come to mind.

It could be your father.

It could be your mother.

It could be your current or ex-husband, wife, boyfriend, or girlfriend.

It could be God.

It could be you.

Whoever it is, feel anger toward that person, and on a scale of 1 to 10, with 10 being highest, build your anger toward that person up to a level 6.

Hold it there for a minute or so and then build your anger toward that person up to a level 8.

Hold your anger toward that person at level 8 for a minute or two, and then push it all the way up to level 10.

Feel intense, level-10 anger towards that person and hold it. In a couple of minutes your anger will start to subside. You'll feel a gradual softening; a slight slipping away, and then your anger will be gone. At that point, take a few deep breaths and think about the person you felt such anger toward. With that person in mind, think about forgiving them.

I know it's hard. I know it's painful. But do it anyway. Take baby steps if you have to, but don't give up. Try to feel real forgiveness for that person. Take a full five minutes or longer here. This is an important step in healing your body.

I've known people who had ugly red acne bumps all over their face for weeks and weeks try the exercise above. Within two days, their skin was completely clear. When you work on releasing anger and practicing forgiveness, amazing things happen.

A Final Word on Forgiveness

We've spoken quite a bit about the need for forgiveness. If it's a new topic for you, give it some serious thought. Most of us have more than one person we need to forgive, so the sooner we start, the better. With all the forgiveness you're now practicing don't forget to forgive the most important person of all: yourself.

It's easy to put ourselves down. When you grow up and are constantly told, "You're stupid", "you're ugly", "you'll never amount to anything", and similar things, it's easy to self-criticize and self-hate. It's easy to believe the messages we receive as children.

How many times have you told yourself, "How could I be so stupid?" How many times have you lowered your head and mentally kicked yourself for something you said or did?

If you're like me, you've done both of the above thousands of times.

It's easy for a person filled with self-criticism and low self-worth to manifest illness. All that negativity creates tremendous toxicity in the body. So be easy and gentle on yourself. Tell yourself you did the best you could with the information you had at the time.

If you hurt somebody else, apologize to that person. If you stole something from somebody, make restitution and give it back. If the person is dead, make restitution to their closest surviving relative. You don't have to explain all the details, just tell the relative that you owed the deceased person money and would like to pay it back. If you stole something from a store or business, mail it back. You can do that anonymously. If you stole someone's time or love apologize to them.

Finally, don't forget to ask God to forgive you.

Chapter Six

The Amazing Power of Sunlight

How important is sunlight? Very important. Sunlight is one of the greatest tools at your disposal for creating a healthy and strong body. The key, though, is not to wear makeup, sunscreen or sunglasses. Let the healing rays of the sun lovingly touch your skin. Start with five minutes a day and gradually increase up to fifteen or twenty minutes a day.

The best times to sunbathe are early in the morning from 6-8 AM, and early in the evening from 5-7 PM. At those times, you get the cooling rays of the sun.

Without sunlight, all life on the planet would die. Think about that for a moment and then ask yourself if you really want to spend all of your time locked up indoors?

Sunlight boosts your immune system and will help clear toxicity out of your body.

Sunlight decreases stress and is great for healing depression. It's almost impossible to feel depressed when you're under the warm, healing rays of the sun. Have you ever wondered why people get depressed when it rains? It's because they can't see the sun or feel its warmth on their skin.

Sunlight is excellent for your vision. If you wear glasses or contacts, spend some time walking around outside without them. You'll notice something amazing. Your vision will begin to clear up. You'll also notice that you can see much better outside in the sun than inside.

Have you ever heard the expression "eagle eye"? It means a person with excellent vision, and it comes from the fact that eagles have excellent eyesight from flying high in the sky with their eyes exposed to the sun. When an eagle swoops down to pluck a fish from the sea their eyes are exposed to the reflection of sunlight off the water.

Sunlight played a huge factor for me in healing astigmatism and improving my vision from 20/800 to 20/60.

I'm using the sun now to improve my vision even more and I expect to reach 20/40 vision sometime over the next few months.

Sunlight is a great source of Vitamin D, an essential nutrient.

Sunlight is a win-win situation. It produces amazing benefits with zero negative effects.

If you are able to expose your entire body to the sun, go for it. If not, don't worry. Just go for a stroll in the early morning or late afternoon and let the sun caress your skin. You'll feel so much better.

Chapter Seven

Sleep Like a King

Sleep is essential when it comes to healing the body from illness. Tissue growth and repair occurs when you sleep and only when you sleep. It actually occurs during the REM (Rapid Eye Movement) phase of sleeping. REM sleep is when you are dreaming and the more you sleep, the more of the REM phase you experience. During the REM phase of sleeping, your body repairs, recharges, revitalizes, and grows.

That's where the expression "beauty sleep" comes from. The more a person sleeps, the more their skin revitalizes and beautifies. Simply put, the more you sleep, the healthier you are and the better you look.

HGH (Human Growth Hormone) is released primarily when you sleep. HGH promotes tissue repair and skin rejuvenation. If you want HGH to do its part in healing your body, be sure to get plenty of sleep.

For athletes reading this, be aware that muscle growth only occurs when you sleep. Your muscles don't grow when you are awake and they don't grow when you are exercising; they grow when you are sleeping. If you're working out, you want to be sure and get lots of sleep.

For guys, sleep is a natural alternative to steroids. In fact, old-time bodybuilding coaches used to recommend sleeping after a workout. They called it a "muscle nap" and the prescription was: workout, consume nutritious protein, and take a nap. That's not always practical in the real world, but if you can do it, why not? The truth is the more you sleep, the faster your muscles grow and the quicker your entire body will heal from any illness you have.

Personally, I function best with ten hours of sleep a night. You might need a little more or a little less. If you are experiencing an adverse reaction to the jab or from shedding, you may need between nine and twelve hours of sleep a night until you are healed.

When you sleep is almost as important as how much. There are certain growth processes that occur in the body from 10 PM to 2 AM that don't occur at any other time, and they only take place when you are sleeping, not when you are awake. So you have to be asleep during those hours in order to benefit.

There are other processes that occur from 2 AM to 6 AM. You have to be asleep during those hours for those growth processes to occur. They won't happen if you're awake.

In order to give your body all of the ammunition it needs to heal it's important for you to be in bed and sleeping every night from 10 PM to 6 AM. Even better would be to sleep from 9 PM to 7 AM.

Did you know that sleep deprivation is a form of torture? It's true. If you want to drive a person crazy, the easiest way to do that is to deprive that person of sleep.

Today, almost the entire population of the world is chronically sleep-deprived. Not to the extreme that would be labeled torture, but certainly enough to create disease in the body, and certainly enough to prevent the body from operating at peak efficiency.

Sleep helps with depression. There's no better way to escape your troubles than sleep. Life got you down? Try taking a nap. You'll feel much better when you wake up.

If you have trouble falling asleep, here's a great tip: try eliminating all sound for thirty minutes before you go to bed. By that, I mean no talking, no music, no television, no sound at all. Your mind will quiet down considerably and you'll find it easy to nod off and enjoy a restful night's sleep.

Also, make sure your bed is comfortable and your room is quiet. If your neighbors are noisy and refuse to quiet down, you have two choices: you can move or you can buy a $20 box fan made by Lasko.

Place the fan near your bed and aim it at the wall so it's not blowing all over you. Your purpose in buying the fan is to create ambient noise. The quiet whir of the fan will do that.

Hopefully, it will be loud enough to drown out your neighbors.

If you have trouble keeping light out of your bedroom, invest in an inexpensive sleep mask. Your body will thank you. Remember, your body grows, repairs, and regenerates while you are sleeping.

Modern life is difficult, so it might not be possible for you to always get the proper amount of sleep. If that's the case with you, do the best you can.

No one ever gets it right all the time, so take comfort knowing that a little improvement is better than no improvement.

Chapter Eight

Honesty is the Best Policy

We live in a world of lies.

Doctors lie to their patients. Teachers lie to their students. Governments lie to their citizens. And television newscasters lie to everyone.

And then we wonder why everyone is sick.

In fact, you could make an argument that the reason why so many people are sick is because they are constantly lying. They lie to their family and friends; they lie to their customers and co-workers; and most of all they lie to themselves—by claiming they don't lie!

What part does honesty play in your body's health? A very large part.

Every time we lie, every time we perform a dishonest act, every time we give truth to a lie in any way (such as agreeing with a lie, giving public support to a lie, or refusing to expose a lie), we weaken our immune system.

You can prove this to yourself with simple kinesiology. Kinesiology is a form of muscle testing that acts as an instant lie detector. Unlike the polygraph tests administered by law enforcement, kinesiology is 100% accurate. It can also be used to determine whether a product, person or place is beneficial to you or not.

Make a truthful statement while using kinesiology to test your muscle's ability to resist and you'll see that your body's response is strong. Then test the same muscle while making a false statement and watch how weak the body becomes.

Now imagine the damage that's being done to a person's immune system when they choose to live a dishonest life, week by week, day by day, hour by hour. It's happening all around us.

One of the worst lies of all is the adult to child lie. There's the child, wide-eyed with innocence and looking for answers, and then there's the adult, usually a parent or teacher, lying through their teeth by repeating what they saw on television.

Granted, some of these parents and teachers are ignorant of the lies they spew. They actually believe in the hoaxes they see on television, including the virus hoax. However, in this new world we all live in, ignorance is no longer an excuse. We all have a duty to learn and report the truth.

What does all of this mean for us?

Simply put, in order for your body to heal, in order to reverse the side effects of the COVID-19 vaccine or to protect yourself from shedding, you must begin living a totally truthful life. Failure to do so could severely retard your progress.

If you're sick and suffering from an adverse reaction to the Trump vaccine, then it's imperative to first admit to yourself that you were fooled and that the entire virus narrative is a hoax. This is an important step so don't overlook it.

To seek to heal yourself on one hand, while clinging to a lie on the other, makes your chances of recovery from illness very slim. Those that took the jab, became crippled or paralyzed from it, and now claim they would do it all over again will never become well.

There's no shame in admitting you're been conned. When I was in grade school, high school and college, I believed every word of nonsense my teachers told me. Looking back, it was a non-stop litany of lies, but I bought it. I bought all of it.

As an adult, realizing what happened, I had two choices. I could remain like most people, afraid to admit when they make a mistake, and continue believing all the lies. Or I could act as an adult should and admit to myself that I'd been conned, taken advantage of, sold a bill of goods. I chose the latter course, and as a famous poet once said, "It has made all the difference."

Refusal to admit a mistake, to admit to yourself that someone has lied to you and that you were wrong to believe them, stems from pride. Pride is one of the seven capital sins, along with covetousness, lust, anger, gluttony, envy and sloth.

Some say pride is the greatest of all sins, because it is the summit of self-love and is directly opposed to submission to God. As such, they say it is the sin most hated by God and the one He punishes most severely.

In today's world we are bombarded with hoaxes on a daily basis. Anyone who falls for one of these hoaxes and refuses to admit it is guilty of the sin of pride.

Follow the Advice of Jacinta from Fatima

Like everything else, living a totally truthful life is simple, but not easy. The easiest way to proceed is to follow the advice given by little Jacinta of Fatima when she said, "Always tell the truth, even when it is hard."

(Jacinta was one of three seers at Fatima, where the Miracle of the Sun took place. The Miracle of the Sun is known as one of the greatest miracles in the history of the world, certainly the greatest miracle since the Resurrection. To learn more about Fatima and the Miracle of the Sun, I recommend reading the books *Our Lady of Fatima*, *The Crusade of Fatima*, and *The Impostor Sister Lucy*.)

For many people, the most difficult part of living a totally truthful life is admitting that they lie. So they won't do it.

Instead, they continue to lie by claiming they live an honest life. Let's see just how honest they are.

Charging too much for a product, service, housing or rent is a form of lying.

People who are guilty of such a lie will immediately draw themselves up and claim that such a statement is not true. They'll say they are merely charging "what they are worth" or charging "fair market value." But that is just another lie.

False or misleading advertising is a form of lying.

Pushing drugs, along with unnecessary surgery, or harmful radiation treatments while calling yourself a doctor is a form of lying.

Teaching fake history in a classroom is a form of lying.

Donning a face mask under the guise of a fake pandemic is a form of lying.

The mask-wearer didn't concoct the lie himself, but he is giving truth to the lie, and doing so in a public manner. Thus he is helping to spread a lie.

To better understand this, consider a movie or theatrical play. You have actors playing leading parts and you have actors playing extras. Both have a duty to suspend the disbelief of the viewing public. Both are responsible for the success of the production. The mask-wearer is akin to the extra. He is not playing a major role, but his participation is necessary for the success of the production.

What about those who don't know any better? The teacher regurgitating data from the school's textbook, the newscaster reading from a prompt, the mask-wearer who actually believes he's doing the right thing ... What about them?

Ignorance might work for them in a court of law with a sympathetic jury. Maybe. But their higher self–their conscience, if you will–knows the truth, and their body will react in the same way as it would if they knew they were telling a lie. Their immune system will weaken and they will be more likely to become ill.

Not fair, you say?

Perhaps. But ignorance is a form of dishonesty. Ignorance exists only because people are too lazy, too indifferent, or too stupid to seek the truth.

There is no escaping the truth. There's no escaping God's law. A person is either telling the truth or they are lying. There is no middle ground. There is no relative truth.

Each of us has an obligation, a duty, to learn the truth and to expose falsehoods and lies. Those who turn their back on reality, who turn their nose up at facts and ignore truthful evidence, because reality, facts and evidence make them uncomfortable, are doing a tremendous disservice to themselves and to society.

They hurt themselves, by weakening their immune system and they hurt society by contributing to the dumbing-down and general stupidity of the world.

Chapter Nine

Dealing with Depression

If you're feeling ill due to an adverse reaction to the Trump vaccine, or from exposure to shedding from someone who is vaccinated, then chances are you're also depressed.

Well, I've got good news for you: You're not alone and help is right around the corner.

The first step in healing depression is to realize that it's not your fault. What you're feeling is nothing more than your body's natural reaction to living in an unnatural society. Your depression is normal and there are millions more who share your sentiments. Indeed, with all the stupidity and oppression occurring today, almost everyone is depressed.

Our country was founded on religious and moral principles. That's a documented fact and it's embedded in the DNA of all Americans. It's no mystery that as our nation has drifted further and further away from its moral foundation, depression and mental illness has skyrocketed. A flower cut from its roots will wither and die. Our country is that flower.

We have replaced religion with consumerism, and replaced morality with victimhood. From a country founded on freedom and individualism, we have devolved into one that fosters tyranny and dependence on government. If you're not wearing the latest fashion, using the latest gadget, sporting the latest tattoo, obsessed with the latest drivel to come out of Hollywood, or wearing a face mask, then there's something wrong with you.

Did you know that virtually all women's magazines, as well as the vast majority of ads, commercials, and television shows, are purposely designed to lower the self-esteem of their readers? It's the same with ads, commercials and television shows aimed at women, and it's done in order to keep them reading, buying, and watching those very same magazines, products, and television shows.

Happy and successful people tend to shop less and save their money. Most of them are too busy to read women's magazines or watch television.

On the other hand, sad, depressed, and lonely people are forever chasing, forever shopping, and forever spending. It's all part of the game.

Our political leaders, with extremely few exceptions, are a disgrace and downright traitorous.

Our culture and our art, which used to elevate both men and women, now degrade them.

Our schools, which used to teach character development and how to think, now teach anything but.

The family unit, once considered sacred in our society, is now targeted for destruction.

Just as children become distraught and physically ill when their mother and father fight and abandon their duty as parents, so do adults become ill when their country loses its way and abandons its principles.

If you're riled up right now, don't be. The mere fact that you're reading this is a clear indication that you possess above average intelligence and sensitivity. Here are some proven and practical steps you can take right now to lighten your mood and heal your depression:

Resolve to live your life according to the moral principles our country was founded on: God, family, and freedom.

I realize that's a revolutionary concept in today's America, but it is absolutely essential if you truly want to heal your depression.

If you have children, then this step is even more important. Our country's education system is going to teach your children the exact opposite of everything written here. It's up to you to teach them character and morality, and the best way to do that is through your own example.

Feed your body correctly. Get off all sugar, junk food, and processed food. Study the work and health discoveries of Dr. Weston Price. He was the first and only scientist to discover the optimum diet for humans to consume.

What you feed your mind is just as important as what you feed your body. Read positive books and articles. Associate with positive people. And here's a radical suggestion: read the New Testament Bible for fifteen minutes a day.

Listen to classical music. It might take a little while to get used to, but once you do, you'll wonder how you ever got along without it.

Get out in the sun more. No plant or animal that lives above ground can survive without the sun, including you.

Stand and sit straight, and practice looking up. It's impossible to feel depressed while looking up, especially if you're looking up at the bright blue sky.

Laugh more. Humor is essential to life. Unfortunately, most humor today consists of ridicule and scorn. Get back to humor that celebrates life.

Praise others whenever possible. Looking for the best in others will bring out the best in you.

Avoid television like the plague. This might be the most important suggestion of all. Television is a means of control, meant to control you. It consists of programs, designed to program your mind. Say no to the hypnotist in the corner. This is especially essential if you have children.

Vote for political candidates who share your belief in God, family, and freedom. Realize that voting for any candidate who supports abortion is a grave sin. Do you really want to risk eternal damnation?

Save money on a regular basis. The amount you save is less important than the habit of regular saving. You'll feel so much better as your savings accumulate.

Thank God for all the blessings in your life. It's impossible to be depressed when you're feeling thankful.

If you're sad because you never achieved your dreams; never reached the pinnacle of success you hoped for; never acquired the money, the fame, the beautiful soul mate you longed for all your life, perish the thought.

Those are worldly pursuits that don't add up to a hill of beans when it comes to achieving the ultimate prize: Heaven.

Where are the great war-mongers of the past, Churchill, Stalin, Lincoln, FDR, Alexander the Great, Genghis Khan and others? Rotting in the grave.

Where are the great movie stars and entertainers of the past? Rotting in the grave.

Where will all of the stars, celebrities and so-called influencers of today be in only a handful of years? Rotting in the grave.

"Thou art dust and to dust thou shalt return."

Focus your time here on earth with acquiring the only thing worth possessing, a future in Heaven, and rejoice in the fact that you still have time remaining to achieve that.

Chapter Ten

Dealing with Dopes

Dealing with dopes is a necessary evil when it comes to healing. And the more successful and pronounced your healing is, the more dopes you'll have to deal with.

When I speak of dopes, I'm not talking about the ignorant or the uneducated. In fact, education has nothing to do with it. The biggest dopes in the world today are doctors, dentists, nurses, health professionals, lawyers, journalists, reporters, media people, teachers, academic professionals, and the like. Plenty of education in that group.

I'm talking about the willfully blind. Those who purposely ignore facts and evidence that run counter to their belief system. And who has been more adamant in ignoring facts and evidence and keeping the virus hoax alive than the people in the professions listed above?

How can you tell if someone is a dope? Well, if they believe in the hoax, that's a sign.

If they believe natural healing doesn't work, that's another sign.

The best advice I can offer for dealing with dopes is don't. Don't deal with them. At best, you'll be wasting your time. At worst, you'll only make them hate you more.

Don't trick yourself into trying to discover the motivation behind their beliefs and behavior. There isn't any other than abject fear of change.

Don't expend brain cells wondering why they're so stupid. You'll never come up with a satisfactory answer other than this: when a person's livelihood depends upon a system of lies, it's very hard to get them to acknowledge the truth.

So leave the dopes alone. Don't socialize with them, don't interact with them. Leave them in their own little minds.

What if you're a businessperson and you have dopes for customers? In that case you'll have to decide what's more important, trying to educate them or keeping their business.

It's pretty much an either-or situation, because dopes hate being educated. In fact, there's nothing a dope detests more than learning the truth and being forced to change their thinking. If you try to educate them, they'll likely take their business elsewhere.

I have plenty of dopes as customers. But then in my case, they know exactly what they're getting when they buy one of my books. Still, many of them come back for more.

Some of them come back, because they secretly believe the same things I do; they believe the truth. But they can't quite come around to admitting it to themselves, because their programming is so strong. There's hope for these people. Not much, but some.

Others come back because they're addicted to outrage and anger and the truth that I present gives them plenty of both. What they fail to realize is the immense harm they're doing to their own bodies. Many of them have a long list of ailments that will never heal due to their self-hatred.

If you're married to a dope, that's tough. I really don't know how to advise you. Divorce is a sin and an affront to God, so that's out of the question. You'll just have to do the best you can.

Other family members who happen to be dopes can be ignored gracefully. The same with friends.

What you're going to find is that most people, the vast majority of the human race, are dopes. It's a sad, but true situation. By no means should you dumb yourself down to fit in. On the contrary, continue to seek knowledge and discovery of the truth. After all, two dopes don't make a smart person.

Have patience and do the best you can. Believe me, I feel for you. I know exactly what you're going through. I'm dealing with dopes all day long.

Chapter Eleven

My Personal Protection Plan from Shedding

It would be wonderful if everyone who took the jab would choose to self-quarantine for six months to a year in order not to harm others with shedding. But we all know that will never happen.

Therefore, my first step in avoiding the negative effects of shedding is to avoid contact with anyone who is vaccinated. That's difficult for two reasons.

First, because I have friends who took the jab that I like to see at times. And second, because in most cases it's hard to tell who has or has not been jabbed.

So far I have not experienced anything negative from being around my friends, but you never know. The possibility is always there, so I take some preventive measures which I'll discuss in a moment. As far as dating anyone who has been vaxxed, I would not recommend it. Unless and until we know exactly what is in the vaccine that's causing so many to die or become ill, it's simply too dangerous; like playing Russian roulette with your life. No date is worth it. Engaging in romance or a relationship with anyone who is vaxxed is one place where any reasonable person has to draw the line.

If I was married and my wife chose to take the jab, it would be the end of any physical contact between us. Of course, if I was married, I would never allow my wife to take the jab in the first place.

What if you don't know someone's status and whether they took the jab or not? In that case, my motto is "when in doubt, stay out."

If you don't know a person's vaccine status and they're not willing to tell you (or they do tell you, but you don't believe them), then why put your health and your life at risk? If that means cutting your social life down in half or even more, so be it. Would you rather be healthy and home by yourself, or sick and ill and fighting for your life in a hospital? (By the way, if the events of the last two years haven't made it clear to you, a hospital is the last place you want to be when you are ill.)

Earlier I mentioned two herbs: Echinacea and Cayenne. I make sure to keep both of them stocked at all times. Cayenne is terrific for circulation and the heart. With so many people suffering from blood clots and heart ailments from the vax and others suffering from shedding, it's an essential herb for me. I use a liquid formula added to water.

Echinacea does a super job of boosting the immune system and increasing the amount of T-cells in the blood. I consider it another must-have for this scary world we live in.

Vitamin C is another item I keep in stock.

I juice daily, usually celery, but if I spend any time around a vaccinated person then as soon as I get home, I begin juicing organic cucumbers and I don't stop until I feel my body has replenished whatever the encounter took out of me.

I follow the dietary guidelines we outlined earlier, avoiding everything on the verboten list.

I read positive and uplifting books.

I try to help and educate people whenever the opportunity arises.

Most important of all, I follow the advice in the next chapter.

Chapter Twelve

The Best Advice I Can Give You

It's taken me awhile, but I've finally come to realize that most, if not all, of the illness we experience in our lives is sent to us from God.

It's sent to get our attention; to make us sit up and take notice. It's done individually and also on a mass scale, such as we're seeing now with so many people dying or becoming ill from the Trump vaccine.

Why would God do that?

Because we're not living our lives the way He wants us to and illness is the only thing that will get our attention.

Consider your own case. Are you truly living your life the way God wants you to?

Really?

Are you participating in any kind of behavior that would make God frown and shake His head? Are you participating in any kind of behavior that you would be embarrassed of or ashamed to admit to in His presence? Maybe that's why you're ill.

Here's an important question: What would your life be like if you weren't ill? If you weren't suffering an adverse reaction to the Trump vaccine or from shedding, would you be engaged in some form of sinful behavior?

Would you be carrying on your life, blissfully ignorant of the path God wants you to take?

Would you be aligned with His one true church, traditional Catholicism?

Think about those things.

Does it make sense now why God may have allowed you to become ill in order to get your attention?

The illness you're suffering and that you think is so horrible might turn out to be the very thing that keeps you from committing mortal sin and going to hell when you die.

But I'm a Nice Person!

When I first considered the concept of God sending us wake-up calls, I thought, "That can't be happening to me. After all, I'm a nice person."

It took me a long time to realize that maybe I wasn't so nice. Dating and sleeping with girls, no matter how "nice" I treated them, wasn't only a grave sin on my part, it was making others complicit in my behavior and damning their souls as well. It was then that I realized being a nice person doesn't count for much in Heaven.

Millions of nice people commit sins of lust every day.

Millions of nice people commit sins of omission every day by tolerating other people's sins of lust.

Millions of nice people are complicit in one of the worst sins of all—murder—by voting for pro-abortion politicians.

Millions of nice people are causing death and serious illness to millions of other nice people by participating in the current virus hoax.

These are all very nice people.

They say "please" and "thank you."

They welcome you into their homes, serve you coffee and tea and ask how you are doing, smiling sweetly all the while.

And yet, they are all horrible sinners.

When you really think about it, being a nice person has to be pretty low in God's pecking order.

After all, it seems like the people who call themselves nice and think themselves nice are the ones causing almost all of the harm in the world today. Could the virus hoax be succeeding without their support?

At least the evil-doers of the world are clear in their agenda. Most of them, anyway. The so-called nice people hide behind a veneer of manners and etiquette. They commit their sins under a cloak of human compassion.

When you think about it, it becomes obvious that a not-so-nice person (gruff, unsmiling, maybe even impolite) who loves God and honors Him by obeying the Ten Commandments is far more likely to go to Heaven than a nice person who breaks even just one Commandment.

In Hollywood, where I lived and worked for many years, I met and socialized with dozens of movie stars, television stars, talk-show hosts, and celebrities of all sorts. They were all very nice people. They were all exceedingly friendly. And yet they were all notorious sinners on their way to hell. Some of them have since died and are burning in hell right now.

Analyzing my own life, I thought back to every illness, every ache and pain I've ever experienced and I realized that, yes, all of these illnesses were wake-up calls from God.

In every case, there was something going on with me at the time that wasn't in alignment with God's wishes. In every case, the illness was sent to me either as a wake-up call to stop committing a particular sin, or as a preemptive strike to prevent me from committing a future sin. And here's the kicker: throughout all of those times, I considered myself a nice person.

How about you?

What's going on in your life that may have caused you to experience an adverse reaction to the Trump vaccine or from exposure to shedding?

Take some time to think about this.

If a thought or idea popped into your head while you were reading these words, write it down. The truth will slowly dawn on you.

Your Life's Purpose

What is your purpose?

Why are you here?

Do you ever think about those things?

Most people believe the purpose of life is to follow their dreams. They believe that because it's what they've been told by well-meaning parents and teachers. Nothing could be further from the truth.

The purpose of life isn't to "follow your dreams." Anyone who tells you that is an idiot. The purpose of life is to use our time here on earth to honor God and prepare our souls to enter Heaven.

If you died today would go to Heaven?

Really?

The sad truth, according to all available evidence—and, yes, we do have evidence—is that very few people ever make it to Heaven. Less than one percent. The vast majority end up burning in the fires of hell for all eternity.

Think about that for a moment. Now does it make sense to you why God might have sent you an illness in order to get your attention?

Most people refuse to listen to God unless and until they are facing some sort of crisis, usually a health crisis. If a crisis is the only way that God can get a person's attention, then what do you expect Him to do? Of course, He's going to send that person a crisis in order to get their attention and possibly save their soul.

Give this matter some thought. If you can put your finger on the reason why God might be sending you an illness in order to get your attention, then you're halfway home to healing it.

When was the last time you prayed?

When was the last time you asked for spiritual guidance?

If it's been a long time, or if you've never prayed for spiritual guidance, maybe this is a good time to do so.

The Absolute Best Advice I Can Give You

What I'm going to say next will anger some people. And truth be told, I would be more popular and sell more books if I didn't include it, but your wellbeing is worth more to me than popularity or money. As I told you at the beginning, this book is different.

The absolute best advice I can give you is to embrace the traditional (pre-Vatican II) Catholic Church. You can take or reject that as you see fit. However, before rejecting it, I would suggest you at least investigate it. To reject traditional Catholicism without investigation is the epitome of stupidity.

I recommend traditional Catholicism because it is necessary for salvation and also because the Catholic Church

81

is the only religion in the world with a long history of documented miracles, including miracles of healing. Sight restored to the blind. Mobility restored to the crippled. Life restored to the dead. It's all there, but only in the Catholic Church.

Now when I say the Catholic Church, I mean the *true* Catholic Church, the pre-Vatican II Church that existed publicly up until the 1960s, and still exists today in small pockets.

What we see coming out of Rome today is not the Catholic Church. In fact, it's the complete opposite. It's the same with all of the schools, hospitals and church buildings today that call themselves Catholic. They are not Catholic and they do not represent the true Catholic Church. They represent a counterfeit church.

A lot of people get confused by that. They see what has happened over the last 60 years: the succession of wicked anti-Popes, the enormous sex scandals, the corruption coming from Rome, and they say, "Wait a second. How can all this corruption, all this scandal, all this evil that I see coming from the Catholic Church represent the true church of Jesus Christ?"

The answer is they don't represent the true church of Jesus Christ, because they are not part of the true Catholic Church. They represent a counterfeit church. The true Catholic Church was infiltrated and subverted by Communists almost a century ago.

Have you ever seen a counterfeit twenty dollar bill? At first glance, it looks just like the real thing. But take a closer look and it's clear that the bill is phony. And when you take a real close look, the fakery becomes so obvious that you wonder how you were ever fooled in the first place.

The same thing happens when you look at the counterfeit church that today pretends to be Catholic. Take a real close look and the fakery becomes so obvious that you wonder how anyone was ever fooled to begin with.

It's just like the virus hoax. In order to see the truth, it's necessary to leave emotions out of the equation and apply only facts, logic, and evidence. Most people are not able or willing to do that.

At this point in time, it should be clear to you that most people—well over 90% of the population—make their decisions about life and justify their actions based on emotions, not on facts and evidence. You might think I'm exaggerating just slightly. Trust me, I'm not. If anything, the actual figure is probably higher than 90% of the population.

When it comes to the subject at hand—the Communist subversion and takeover of the Catholic Church and the creation of a counterfeit church—the deception is so huge, so monstrous, and so evil that hundreds of millions of people refuse to acknowledge it. They demonstrate the same mindset as those who were duped into believing the virus hoax. Many of them have been fooled into believing both, the virus hoax and the counterfeit church.

These folks are so frightened of the truth that the majority of them refuse to even look at the evidence. In fact, just mentioning this subject causes their hands to shake and the spittle to fly from their mouths. That's how frightened they are of the truth.

As Saint Thomas Aquinas said, "The greatest charity one can do to another is to lead him to the truth."

As for me, I'm an evidence guy. I learned long ago that opinions are a cheap commodity, but evidence is something else. Evidence reigns supreme. I always follow the evidence, wherever it leads me, and let the chips fall where they may. Here's some evidence you might want to consider: the Catholic Church is the only religion in the world with tens of thousands of documented miracles.

From hard physical evidence that you can see with your own eyes and touch with your own hands, such as the Shroud of Turin (the burial cloth of Jesus Christ) and the Blessed Virgin's miraculous imprint of herself on Juan Diego's tilma at Guadalupe, Mexico in 1530, to the 70,000 eye witnesses who were present at the Miracle of the Sun at Fatima, Portugal in 1917, the Catholic Church has it all: saints whose bodies defy all science and physics by not decomposing after their death, miraculous healings, documented cases of saints raising the dead, documented cases of bilocation in which priests and mystics appear at two or more places at the same time, miraculous battlefield victories against incredible odds as high as 10,000 to 1, and on and on and on; literally tens of thousands of documented miracles within the true Catholic Church.

Meanwhile, all of the other religions of the world combined, numbering in the hundreds, or even the thousands, do not contain one single documented miracle among them. Not one. As I said, I side with the evidence.

A Story of My Own

I've told you already that as a child I was nearly blind with 20/800 vision and astigmatism. I wore thick bifocal glasses almost half an inch wide all through grade school and then contact lenses in high school. Without my glasses or contacts, I couldn't see a thing. Anything beyond six inches in front of me was a blur. Of course, every eye doctor I spoke with told me my vision was incurable and impossible to improve, so naturally I believed them.

As an adult I made a decision to heal my eyesight and have since improved my daytime vision from 20/800 to 20/60. Most of my improvement has come in the last two months and today I was walking down the sidewalk when suddenly my vision became so crystal clear it literally took my breath away. For the first time in my life I saw the world in rich detailed color. It was beyond 20/20 vision and I felt as if I had just been born; as if life for me had just begun at that very moment. It lasted about ten minutes.

Keep all that in mind and consider this: Earlier in this book, I mentioned Fatima and the Miracle of the Sun. I've known about Fatima for years, but only in the last four months have I really gotten into it, reading close to a dozen books on the subject and studying it in depth.

Could there be a connection between my study and newfound knowledge of Fatima and the Miracle of the Sun and the recent and dramatic improvement in my vision? An improvement that dozens of doctors and optometrists all told me was impossible?

Is it possible that as my eyes have been opened to the miracle and message of Fatima, that God, in turn, has opened my eyes here on Earth?

Or is it, as the frightened ninnies will say, all just a coincidence?

You decide.

Read These Books

I recommend you read the book *Outside the Catholic Church There is Absolutely No Salvation* by Brother Peter Dimond. You can find that book at several locations on the internet, and also at this specific website: www.MostHolyFamilyMonastery.com

If you can't afford to buy the book, which sells for around twenty bucks, then visit the website and read all of their free information. Watch their free videos. Immerse yourself in the truth.

Now if you're really courageous; if you're the absolute bravest of the brave, the strongest of the strong; afraid of no man and willing to do whatever it takes to achieve eternal glory, then read the book *Preparation for Death* by Saint Alphonsus Liguori.

I must warn you, it's not for the squeamish. You'll need the strength of Sampson to even begin reading it, and most people are too cowardly and too weak to do even that. It's that same cowardice and that same weakness that prevents the vast majority of men and women from resisting sin and leads to their being condemned to eternity burning in the fires of hell. All because they are too afraid to read a book or visit a website.

What about you?

Where do you stand?

You want to heal yourself from adverse reactions to the Trump vaccine or from exposure to shedding? You got it. Just follow the recommendations in this book.

You want to go to Heaven? You got that too. Just follow the true Catholic faith. It won't be easy, but then no one goes to Heaven without suffering. Better to suffer here on earth, than in the afterlife.

And don't forget, I'm here to help you. When you bought this book you also purchased my personal support. You can contact me at any time for any reason and I will be happy to help you in any way I can.

God bless you and may we meet again in Heaven.

Thank you very much for buying this book!

If you enjoyed it, please leave a review. Even a short, one-sentence review will help.

If you did not enjoy it, please email me with suggestions to improve the text:

Mikestone114@yahoo.com

Mike Stone is the author of *Based*, a young adult novel about race, dating and growing up in America, and *A New America*, a dark comedy set on Election Day 2016..

A New America

On the most divisive day of the year, in the most racially-charged city in America, recently red-pilled movie producer John Duke is about to learn what political correctness really means: marching with the herd or losing everything, including his family.

5 Stars! "A well-written book of an America gone mad."

5 Stars! "More!! Great read!"

5 Stars! "An exciting well-written novel. The author uses no clichés, his descriptions are original, and as a whole the writing is very creative."

5 Stars! "A fast-paced exciting novel."

5 Stars! "Read it all in one sitting. Had to remind myself it's supposed to be fiction."

5 Stars! "I hope this book is read far and wide, because it is the truth."

5 Stars! "You would never see a book written like this in a mainstream publication."

Made in the USA
Monee, IL
15 August 2022

11712880R00059